LOST

AND

FOUND

A Journey Through Alzheimer's

Kayla S. Brigman

Library of Congress Cataloging-in-Publication Data is available upon request.

ISBN 9798393031800

Cover design by *Arlene van Roosmalen*

Printed in the United States of America

Dedication

This book is dedicated to all those affected by Alzheimer's disease. May it offer a glimpse into the journey of those lost to us, and a reminder of the love and memories that will always be `found within our hearts.

Preface

Alzheimer's disease is a condition that affects millions of people worldwide, and its impact on individuals, families, and society is significant. It is a journey through which the patients and their families experience various emotions, from hope and despair to acceptance and perseverance. "*Lost and Found*" is a book that explores this journey and aims to provide comfort and support to those who are going through this experience.

In this book, the author shares their personal journey with Alzheimer's disease, from the initial diagnosis to the final stages of the illness. Through their experiences, the author illuminates the struggles, challenges, and triumphs of living with Alzheimer's disease. The author also provides practical advice and guidance to caregivers and family members supporting their loved ones with Alzheimer's.

The famous philosopher Jean-Paul Sartre once said, "We are our choices." Similarly, the choices we make when caring for someone with Alzheimer's disease can make all the difference in their quality of life. "*Lost and Found*" encourages caregivers and family members to make informed choices, to be patient and kind, and to seek help when needed.

Latin, the classical language studied for centuries, reminds us of the continuity of human experience. Through our shared experiences of love, loss, and aging, we can connect with others and find comfort and solace in our humanity. "*Lost and Found*" is a testament to this human connection and the resilience of the human spirit.

I hope this book will serve as a source of comfort and inspiration to those who are living with Alzheimer's disease or caring for someone who is. It is a journey that can be challenging and heartbreaking, but it is also a journey that can be filled with love, hope, and moments of joy.

Sincerely,

Kayla S. Brigman

Table of Contents

Introduction

This book is a heartfelt and honest account of one family's experience with Alzheimer's disease. It is a story of loss but also of love and the strength of the human spirit.

In these pages, you will follow along as the author navigates the complex and emotional journey of caring for a loved one with Alzheimer's. From the early warning signs and diagnosis to the daily struggles and triumphs of living with the disease, this book is an intimate and compassionate look at the realities of Alzheimer's.

But "*Lost and Found*" is more than just a story of caregiving. It is also a story of hope and resilience. Through the author's personal struggles and reflections, you will discover how she found meaning and purpose amid arduous circumstances.

Whether you are a caregiver or simply looking for a deeper understanding of this devastating disease, "Lost and Found" will offer you comfort, insight, and the inspiration to find hope in even the darkest times. Thank you for joining me on this journey.

Chapter 1

The Early Warning Signs and Symptoms of Alzheimer's

Myth: *"Alzheimer's disease is a normal aspect of aging that only affects the elderly."*

This myth is not true. While Alzheimer's is more common in older adults, it can also affect younger individuals. It is not a natural part of aging but rather a progressive brain disease that affects memory, thinking, and behavior.

One of the most challenging aspects of Alzheimer's disease is that it tends to develop gradually, often with subtle warning signs that can be easily overlooked or attributed to other causes. However, early diagnosis and treatment are critical for slowing the progression of the disease and improving the quality of life for both the patient and the caregiver.

Some common early warning signs of Alzheimer's include:

1. **Memory Loss That Disrupts Daily Life:**

This form of memory loss can include forgetting important dates or appointments, repeatedly asking for the same information, or struggling to remember familiar names or places.

2. **Difficulty Completing Familiar Tasks:**

This difficulty in completing familiar tasks could be as simple as forgetting the steps involved in a task that the person has done many times before or becoming lost while driving in a familiar area.

3. **Challenges With Planning Or Problem-Solving:**

Challenges with planning or problem-solving could involve difficulties following a recipe, paying bills, or making decisions.

4. **Confusion With Time Or Place:**

Confusion with time or place might include getting lost on a familiar route, forgetting where or how they got there, or misplacing objects in unusual places.

5. **Trouble Understanding Visual Images Or Spatial Relationships:**

Reading, gauging distance, or recognizing changes in color or contrast could all be signs of trouble processing visual imagery or spatial relationships.

6. **New Word-Usage Issues While Speaking Or Writing:**

Problems with speaking or writing words could involve difficulty following or joining a conversation or finding the right word during a conversation.

If you or a loved one are experiencing any warning signs, speaking with a healthcare professional as soon as possible is essential. Early diagnosis can allow for earlier treatment and intervention, which can improve the overall prognosis for the patient.

It is also important to remember that other conditions can cause these symptoms, so a thorough evaluation is necessary to determine the cause.

The Diagnosis: Confirming and Coping with the News

Receiving a diagnosis of Alzheimer's disease can be a devastating and overwhelming experience for both the patient and their loved ones. It is normal to feel a range of emotions, including grief, fear, anger, and denial. It is crucial to allow yourself time to process and cope with the news and to seek support from loved ones, healthcare professionals, and support groups.

The process of receiving a diagnosis of Alzheimer's involves a thorough evaluation by a healthcare professional, including medical history, physical examination, and cognitive and neurological testing. It may also include brain imaging scans and laboratory tests to rule out other potential causes of the symptoms.

If the healthcare professional determines that Alzheimer's is the most likely cause of the symptoms, they will discuss the diagnosis with the patient and their loved ones. It is essential to ask questions and clarify any concerns during this conversation. The healthcare professional can also provide information on treatment options and resources for support.

It is important to remember that a diagnosis of Alzheimer's is not a death sentence. While there is no cure for the disease, there are treatments and interventions that can help slow its progression and improve the quality of life for the patient. Taking care of one's physical and emotional health is also essential, as this can help maintain overall well-being.

Receiving a diagnosis of Alzheimer's can be a difficult and emotional experience, but it is essential to remember that there is support and hope. Lean on loved ones, seek resources and support groups, and care for yourself as you navigate this journey.

The Emotional Rollercoaster: Dealing with Grief and Loss

Caring for a loved one with Alzheimer's can be a deeply emotional experience, as it often involves watching a once vibrant and independent individual decline over time. It is common for caregivers to experience a range of emotions, including grief, sadness, frustration, and anger.

It is essential to allow yourself time and space to process these emotions and to seek support from loved ones and professionals.

Grief is a normal and natural response to loss, and caring for a loved one with Alzheimer's can feel like a series of losses. It can be difficult to watch a loved one struggle with memory loss, changes in communication, and the loss of independence. It is important to allow yourself time to grieve these losses and recognize that feeling a range of emotions is okay.

It is also common for caregivers to feel overwhelmed and stressed as they navigate the challenges of caregiving. Making time for self-care and seeking support from loved ones, friends, and professionals is essential. Support groups can also be valuable, providing a space to connect with others experiencing similar challenges.

Remember that it is okay to feel a range of emotions and that taking care of your emotional well-being is essential. Seek support when you need it, and try to find ways to find joy and meaning amid arduous circumstances.

Chapter 2

Navigating the Healthcare System and Finding the Right Care

Caring for a loved one with Alzheimer's can be overwhelming, especially when navigating the healthcare system. It is vital to advocate for your loved one and do your best to ensure that they receive the best possible care.

Here are a few tips for finding the proper care for a loved one with Alzheimer's:

1. **Start with A Primary Care Physician:** Your loved one's primary care physician can help

coordinate their care and refer them to specialists.

2. **Seek Out Specialists**: Depending on your loved one's needs, they may benefit from seeing specialists such as a geriatrician, neurologist, or psychiatrist.

3. **Explore Treatment Options**: There is a range of treatment options available for Alzheimer's, including medications, behavioral therapies, and non-pharmacological interventions. Discussing the pros and cons of these options with the healthcare team and considering your loved one's specific needs and preferences is essential.

4. **Consider Alternative Therapies**: While there is no cure for Alzheimer's, some alternative treatments, such as music therapy, art therapy, or pet therapy, may help improve the quality of life and reduce stress for the patient and the caregiver.

5. **Learn About Community Resources**: There are many community resources available to help caregivers and loved ones with Alzheimer's, including adult daycare centers, respite care, and home health agencies. Exploring these options and finding what works best for your loved one is essential.

6. **Stay Organized**: Keeping a record of your loved one's medical appointments, medications, and any other important information can be helpful. Staying

organized can help you stay organized and ensure your care is coordinated.

7. **Don't Be Afraid To Ask For Help**: Caregiving for a loved one with Alzheimer's can be overwhelming. It is vital to seek support from loved ones, friends, and professionals when needed.

Navigating the healthcare system can be challenging, but with patience and persistence, you can find the proper care for your loved one with Alzheimer's.

Adjusting to a New Normal: Making Changes at Home and Work

Caring for a loved one with Alzheimer's often requires significant daily routines and responsibilities changes. It is essential to be flexible and adjust to ensure the best care for your loved one. Here are a few tips for making changes at home and work:

1. **Make Safety A Priority**:

As Alzheimer's progresses, your loved one may become more forgetful or confused and at risk for accidents such as falls or fires. It is essential to make the home safe, such as installing grab bars, removing tripping hazards, and ensuring that medications are stored securely.

2. **Simplify Daily Tasks**:

As your loved one's cognitive abilities decline, they may struggle with tasks that were once easy for them. It can be helpful to simplify daily tasks and routines, such as breaking tasks down into smaller steps or using visual cues to help them remember what to do.

3. **Consider Home Modifications:**

Depending on your loved one's needs, you may need to modify the home to accommodate their changing abilities. Using home modifications could include adding ramps or handrails or making other changes to make the home more accessible.

4. **Make Arrangements At Work:**

If you are a caregiver and work outside of the home, it may be necessary to adjust your work schedule or responsibilities. Communicating with your employer about your caregiving responsibilities and exploring options such as flexible work schedules or working from home is essential.

5. **Seek Out Support:**

Caregiving for a loved one with Alzheimer's can be overwhelming. It is crucial to seek help from loved ones, friends, and professionals when needed. Support groups can also be valuable for connecting with others facing similar challenges.

Adjusting to a new normal can be difficult, but with patience, flexibility, and a willingness to seek support, you can find a way to make it work

Self-Care Is Crucial For Caregivers, As Is Caring For Others.

As a caregiver for a loved one with Alzheimer's, it is important to remember to take care of yourself as well. Caregiving can be a demanding and stressful role, and it is essential to prioritize your own physical and emotional well-being.

Here are a few tips for self-care as a caregiver:

1. **Take Breaks:** It is essential to make time for yourself and to take breaks from caregiving

responsibilities. Taking breaks can be as simple as taking a walk or spending time with friends, or it could involve seeking respite care to give you a longer break.

2. **Exercise And Eat Well**: Caring for a loved one with Alzheimer's can be physically and emotionally draining. It is vital to prioritize exercise and healthy eating to help maintain your physical and emotional well-being.

3. **Get Enough Sleep**: Sleep is essential for physical and emotional health. To feel rested and rejuvenated, make sure you receive enough sleep each night.

4. **Seek Out Support**: Caregiving can be isolating, and it is essential to seek support from loved ones, friends, and professionals. Support groups can also be valuable for connecting with others facing similar challenges.

5. **Take Time For Yourself:** Make time for activities that bring you joy and relaxation, whether reading, hobbies, or in nature.

Caring for a loved one with Alzheimer's can be demanding and rewarding, but it is essential to remember to take care of yourself as well. With some self-care, you can be a better caregiver and find the strength to navigate this journey.

Chapter 3

Communication Challenges: Navigating Changes in Speech and Cognition

One of the most challenging aspects of Alzheimer's is how it can affect communication. As the disease progresses, individuals with Alzheimer's may struggle with speech, language, and cognitive skills, making it challenging to communicate their needs and wants.

Here are a few tips for navigating communication challenges as a caregiver:

1. **Be Patient**: It can be frustrating to communicate with a loved one with Alzheimer's, but it is essential to be patient and to allow them time to process and respond.

2. **Use Nonverbal Cues**: Nonverbal cues such as facial expressions, gestures, and touch can be powerful tools for communication. Use these cues to help convey meaning and to connect with your loved one.

3. **Use Simple Language**: As cognitive abilities decline, it can be helpful to use simple language and to speak slowly and clearly. Avoid using complex words or sentences, and repeat yourself as needed.

4. **Use Visual Aids**: Visual aids such as pictures, diagrams, or written words can help convey meaning and for helping your loved one understand what you are saying.

5. **Pay Attention to Body Language**: Your loved one's body language and nonverbal cues can help you understand what they are trying to communicate.

6. **Seek out Speech Therapy**: If you are concerned about your loved one's ability to communicate, it may be helpful to seek out speech therapy. A speech therapist can help develop strategies for improving communication and supporting the patient and the caregiver.

Navigating communication challenges can be difficult, but with patience and persistence, you can find ways to connect with your loved one and help them communicate their needs..

Using Music Therapy to Connect with Loved Ones

Music has the power to connect people in a deep and meaningful way, and it can be especially beneficial for individuals with Alzheimer's. Music therapy involves using music to address the physical, emotional, cognitive, and social needs of individuals with various conditions, including Alzheimer's.

Here are a few ways in which music therapy can be beneficial for individuals with Alzheimer's:

1. **Improves Communication**: Music therapy can help individuals with Alzheimer's improve communication skills by providing a nonverbal way to express emotions and ideas.

2. **Increases Socialization**: Music therapy can help individuals with Alzheimer's connect with others and increase socialization, improving quality of life and reducing feelings of isolation.

3. **Provides a Sense of Control**: As Alzheimer's progresses, individuals may lose control over many aspects of their lives. Music therapy can provide a sense of control and autonomy by allowing individuals to participate in music-making.

4. **Reduces Agitation**: Music has been shown to have a calming effect on individuals with Alzheimer's, and music therapy can help reduce fever and aggressive behavior.

5. **Improves Cognitive Skills**: Music therapy has been shown to improve cognitive skills such as memory, attention, and problem-solving in individuals with Alzheimer's.

Music therapy can be a powerful tool for connecting with loved ones with Alzheimer's and improving their quality of life. If you want to explore music therapy for a loved one with Alzheimer's, working with a trained and certified music therapist is essential. The therapist will work with you and your loved one to develop a customized music therapy plan that meets their needs and goals.

Music therapy can be conducted in various settings, including in the home, healthcare facility, or community setting. It can be performed individually or in a group and involves multiple activities such as singing, listening to music, playing an instrument, or moving to music.

If you are considering music therapy for a loved one with Alzheimer's, it is crucial to keep an open mind and to be willing to try different activities and approaches. What works for one individual may not work for another, and finding the right fit may take some time.

Overall, the power of music can be a valuable tool for connecting with loved ones with Alzheimer's and improving their quality of life. By working with a trained music therapist and being open to trying different approaches, you can find the right fit for your loved one.

The Role of Hobbies and Creativity

Finding joy in the small things can be vital to caring for a loved one with Alzheimer's, as it can provide a sense of purpose and meaning amid difficult circumstances. Hobbies and creative activities can be a valuable way to connect with your loved one and to find joy in the present moment.

Here are a few ideas for incorporating hobbies and creativity into caregiving:

1. Encourage Your Loved One To Pursue Their Interests:

If your loved one enjoyed a particular hobby or activity before their diagnosis, try to find ways to continue participating in that activity. Encouraging your loved one to pursue their interests could be as simple as looking at old photo albums or playing a favorite game.

2. **Explore New Hobbies:**

Trying out new hobbies and activities can be a fun and enriching way to spend time together. Exploring new hobbies could be something as simple as gardening or cooking or something more structured like a painting class.

3. **Encourage Creativity:**

Creativity can take many forms, and finding what works best for your loved one is essential. Encouraging creativity could be something as simple as coloring, drawing, or something more hands-on like sculpture or woodworking.

4. **Seek Out Community Resources:**

Many communities offer classes and activities specifically designed for individuals with Alzheimer's and their caregivers. These can be a great way to connect with others and try new hobbies and activities.

5. **Find Joy In Everyday Activities**:

Hobbies and creative activities don't have to be elaborate or time-consuming. Finding joy in the small things, such as enjoying a beautiful sunset or listening to music together, can bring a sense of meaning and connection.

Hobbies and creative activities can be a valuable way to find joy and meaning while caring for a loved one with Alzheimer's. By encouraging your loved one to pursue their interests and finding joy in the small things, you can create positive and enriching experiences together.

Chapter 4

The Role of Family and Friends in Building a Support System

Caring for a loved one with Alzheimer's can be a challenging and isolating experience, and it is crucial to have a strong support system in place to help navigate the journey. Family and friends can be vital in providing emotional, practical, and financial support for caregivers and loved ones with Alzheimer's.

Here are a few ways in which family and friends can provide support:

1. **Offer Practical Help:**

Many tasks must be done when caring for a loved one with Alzheimer's, and it can be overwhelming for caregivers to manage everything independently. Offering practical help, such as running errands, doing groceries, or helping with housework, can be a valuable way to lighten the load for caregivers.

2. **Provide Emotional Support:**

Caregiving can be emotionally draining, and it is crucial to have a supportive network of loved ones to turn to when things get tough. Simply listening and offering a shoulder to lean on can make a big difference.

3. **Be An Advocate:**

As a caregiver, having someone to advocate for you and your loved one can be helpful.

Becoming an advocate could involve the following:

- Helping to navigate the healthcare system.

- Communicating with professionals.

- Assisting with financial and legal matters.

4. **Take Breaks:**

It is essential for caregivers to take breaks and to have time for themselves. Encourage caregivers to take a break, offer to step in, and provide care while away.

5. **Seek Out Community Resources:**

Many communities offer support groups and other resources for caregivers and loved ones with Alzheimer's. Encourage caregivers to explore these options and seek out support when needed.

Overall, having a strong family and friends support system can be an invaluable resource for caregivers and loved ones with Alzheimer's. Family and friends can make the caregiving journey more accessible by offering practical and emotional support and being an advocate.

The Role of Medications in Managing Alzheimer's

Medications can play a role in managing the symptoms of Alzheimer's and in slowing the progression of the disease. Working with a healthcare professional to determine the best treatment plan for your loved one is essential, as each individual's needs are unique.

Here is a brief overview of the types of medications that may be used to manage Alzheimer's:

1. **Cholinesterase Inhibitors:**

These medications work by increasing the levels of a chemical called acetylcholine, which is essential for memory and cognitive function. The cholinesterase inhibitors donepezil, rivastigmine, and galantamine are other examples.

2. **Memantine:**

This medication works by regulating the activity of a chemical called glutamate, which is involved in learning and memory. Combining memantine with a cholinesterase inhibitor is common practice.

3. **Antidepressants and Antipsychotics:**

You can use these medications to manage symptoms such as depression, anxiety, agitation, or psychosis. It is essential to carefully monitor the use of these medications in individuals with Alzheimer's, as they can have side effects and may not be appropriate for all individuals.

It is important to remember that medications are only one aspect of managing Alzheimer's and should be used with other treatments and interventions, such as behavioral and non-pharmacological interventions.

It is also essential to be aware of the potential side effects of medications and to discuss any concerns with a healthcare professional.

Overall, medications can play a valuable role in managing the symptoms of Alzheimer's. Still, it is essential to work with a healthcare professional to determine the best treatment plan for your loved one.

Choosing the Right Level of Care

As Alzheimer's progresses, caregivers may face the difficult decision of choosing the right level of care for their loved one. Choosing the right level of care can be a challenging and emotional process. It is essential to consider the options carefully and involve the loved one in decision-making as much as possible.

Here are a few factors to consider when choosing the right level of care:

1. **Safety:**

The most important consideration when choosing the right level of care is the safety of your loved one. If your loved one is at risk for accidents or injuries, it may be necessary to consider more intensive levels of care, such as assisted living or nursing home care.

2. **Quality of Life:**

It is also essential to consider the quality of life of your loved one. While more intensive levels of care may provide more structure and support, they may also be more restrictive and offer a different level of independence than home care.

3. **Finances:**

The cost of care is an important consideration, and it is vital to explore all available options and to understand what insurance or other financial resources cover.

4. **Personal Preferences:**

It is crucial to involve your loved one in decision-making as much as possible and to consider their personal preferences and needs.

5. Professional Guidance:

It can be helpful to seek out the guidance of a geriatric care manager or other professional to help evaluate the needs of your loved one and explore the available options.

Levels of Care to Consider

Choosing the right level of care can be difficult, but with careful consideration and professional guidance, you can find the best option for your loved one. Here are a few different levels of care to consider:

1. Home Care:

Home care involves providing care in the home and can include a range of services such as bathing, dressing, medication management, and companionship. A family member, a paid caregiver, or a combination can provide home care.

2. **Assisted Living**:

Assisted living facilities provide a combination of housing, personal care, and health services for individuals who need assistance with activities of daily living. Assisted living facilities typically offer more structure and support than home care but may also be more restrictive and offer a different level of independence.

3. **Nursing Home Care**:

Nursing homes provide 24-hour medical and personal care for individuals who need more support. Nursing homes offer a more structured and supportive environment. Still, they may also be more restrictive and provide a different level of privacy and autonomy than home care or assisted living.

4. **Hospice Care**:

Hospice care is a type of care that is focused on comfort and quality of life for individuals who are in the final stages of a terminal illness.

Hospice care can be provided in various settings, including in the home, hospital, or hospice facility.

Ultimately, the right level of care will depend on the needs and preferences of your loved one. It is crucial to consider the options carefully and involve your loved one in decision-making as much as possible. You can find the best choice for your loved one with careful planning and professional guidance.

Chapter 5

Dealing with Aggression and Behavioral Changes

Dealing with aggression and behavioral changes can be challenging when caring for a loved one with Alzheimer's. As the disease progresses, individuals with Alzheimer's may experience changes in behavior, such as agitation, aggression, and resistance to care. It is important to remember that these behaviors are often a result of the disease and are not intentional.

Below are a few strategies for dealing with aggression and behavioral changes:

1. **Identify The Cause:**

It is essential to identify the cause of the behavior and address any underlying issues such as pain, hunger, or discomfort.

2. **Use Nonverbal Communication:**

Nonverbal communication, such as facial expressions, touch, and body language, can be powerful tools for calming and reassuring a loved one with Alzheimer's.

3. **Provide A Calm Environment:**

A calm and peaceful environment can help reduce agitation and aggression. Providing a quiet environment may involve:

- Reducing noise and distractions.

- Providing comfortable and familiar surroundings.

- Using soothing music or lighting.

4. **Use Positive Reinforcement:**

Positive reinforcement can be an effective way to encourage positive behaviors and discourage negative behaviors. Positive reinforcement may involve praising and rewarding desired behaviors or simply offering a smile and words of encouragement.

5. **Seek Professional Help:**

If aggressive or disruptive behaviors are persistent and difficult to manage, it may be helpful to seek the guidance of a healthcare professional or a behavioral therapist.

Dealing with aggression and behavioral changes can be challenging. Still, with patience and understanding, finding ways to manage these behaviors and provide a supportive and nurturing environment for your loved one is possible.

Important Conversations and Decisions for End-of-Life Planning

End-of-life planning can be complex and emotional, but it is essential to caring for a loved one with Alzheimer's. It is possible to guarantee that your loved one's desires are respected and that they receive the care they seek at the end of life by having open and honest conversations and making decisions in advance.

Here are a few things to consider when it comes to end-of-life planning:

1. **Advance Directives:**

Advance directives are legal documents that outline an individual's preferences for medical treatment at the end of life. These documents can include a living will, which specifies treatment preferences, and a durable power of attorney for healthcare, which designates a person to make medical decisions on behalf of the individual.

2. **End-Of-Life Care Options:**

It is essential to consider the various end-of-life options available, such as hospice care, palliative care, or in-home care. Each option has its benefits and limitations, and it is essential to consider what is best for your loved one carefully.

3. **Finances:**

End-of-life care can be expensive, and it is crucial to understand what is covered by insurance and to make financial plans in advance. Finances may involve exploring options such as long-term care insurance or Medicaid.

4. **Emotional Considerations:**

End-of-life planning can be an emotional and challenging process, and it is vital to allow yourself and your loved one time to process your feelings. It can be helpful to seek out the support of a therapist or a support group.

Overall, end-of-life planning is essential to caring for a loved one with Alzheimer's. By having open and honest conversations and making decisions in advance, you can ensure that your loved one's wishes are respected and that they receive the care they desire at the end of life.

Coping with the Loss of a Loved One

Losing a loved one with Alzheimer's can be a difficult and emotional experience, and it is crucial to allow yourself time to grieve and process your feelings. Here are a few tips for coping with the loss of a loved one:

1. Take Care Of Yourself:

Grief can be physically and emotionally draining, and taking care of yourself during this time is essential. Get enough rest, eat well, and find time for activities that bring you comfort and relaxation.

2. Seek Support:

It can be helpful to seek out the support of loved ones, a therapist, or a support group. Talking about your feelings and connecting with others who are going through a similar experience can be a valuable source of comfort.

3. **Look for Ways to Remember Your Loved One:**

There are many ways to honor and remember a loved one, such as creating a memorial, volunteering, or simply sharing memories with others.

4. **Allow Yourself Time To Grieve:**

Grief is a natural and normal response to loss, and it is crucial to allow yourself time to process your feelings. There is no right or wrong way to grieve; it is essential to be patient and allow yourself to feel your emotions.

5. **Find Ways to Move Forward:**

While allowing yourself time to grieve is crucial, finding ways to move forward and find meaning and purpose in the aftermath of loss is also essential. Finding ways to move forward may involve finding new hobbies or activities or simply finding joy in the small things.

6. **Find Ways To Celebrate Their Life:**

It can be comforting to celebrate the life of your loved one and to remember the joy and meaning they brought to your life. Finding ways to celebrate the life of your loved one could involve:

- Creating a photo album or slideshow.

- Sharing stories and memories with others.

- Simply taking time to reflect on the special moments you shared.

7. **Find Meaning In The Caregiving Journey:**

Caregiving can be a challenging and demanding role, but it can also be a gratifying and meaningful experience. It can be helpful to reflect on the caregiving journey and to find meaning in the time you spend together.

8. **Seek Out Professional Help If Needed:**

It is entirely normal to experience a wide range of emotions after losing a loved one, and it is vital to seek professional help if needed. A therapist or counselor can provide a safe and supportive space to process your feelings and find ways to cope with your loss.

Remember, allowing yourself time to grieve and being patient with yourself as you navigate this challenging experience is essential. It is okay to take things one day at a time and seek support when needed.

Finding Healing and Hope

Grieving the loss of a loved one with Alzheimer's can be a complex and emotional process, but it is also an essential aspect of healing and moving forward. While it is natural to experience a wide range of emotions during this time, finding ways to find healing and hope as you navigate the grieving process is essential.

Here are a few tips for finding healing and hope after the loss of a loved one:

1. Allow Yourself Time To Grieve:

It's critical to give yourself time to grieve and digest your feelings. There is no right or wrong way to grieve, and you must be patient with yourself as you navigate this challenging experience.

2. Find Ways to Remember Your Loved One:

There are many ways to honor and remember a loved one, such as creating a memorial, volunteering, or simply sharing memories with others.

3. Seek Out Support:

It can be helpful to seek out the support of loved ones, a therapist, or a support group. Talking about your feelings and connecting with others who are going through a similar experience can be a valuable source of comfort.

4. Find Meaning In The Caregiving Journey:

Caregiving can be challenging and demanding, but it can also be an advantageous and meaningful experience. It can be helpful to reflect on the caregiving journey and to find meaning in the time you spend together.

5. **Find Joy In The Small Things:**

It can be challenging to find joy and happiness in the aftermath of loss, but finding ways to find meaning and purpose in the small things is important. Finding joy in the small things may involve finding new hobbies or activities or simply finding joy in the beauty of nature or the company of loved ones.

Grieving the loss of a loved one with Alzheimer's can be difficult and emotional, but it is also an opportunity for healing and growth. By allowing yourself time to grieve, finding ways to remember your loved one, and finding joy and meaning in the small things, you can find healing and hope as you move forward.

Remember, it is okay to take things one day at a time and to seek out support when needed. It is also essential to be patient with yourself and to permit yourself to experience a wide range of emotions during this time.

Chapter 6

Lessons Learned and Growth through Alzheimer's

Caring for a loved one with Alzheimer's can be a challenging and demanding experience, but it can also be an opportunity for growth and personal development. Here are a few ways that caring for a loved one with Alzheimer's can lead to personal growth and development:

1. Emotional Growth:

Caring for a loved one with Alzheimer's can be emotionally challenging but can also provide an opportunity for emotional growth. It can teach us empathy, patience, and the importance of self-care.

2. **Personal Growth:**

Caring for a loved one with Alzheimer's can be demanding and require much time and energy. However, it can also lead to personal growth as caregivers learn to prioritize their needs and find balance.

3. **Relationship Growth:**

Caring for a loved one with Alzheimer's can be an opportunity to strengthen relationships with family and friends as caregivers reach out for support and help. It can also be an opportunity to strengthen relationships with the loved one with Alzheimer's as caregivers learn to communicate and connect in new ways.

4. **Appreciation For The Present Moment:**

Caring for a loved one with Alzheimer's can be a reminder to appreciate the present moment and to find joy and meaning in the small things. It can also be an opportunity to learn to relinquish expectations and focus on what is truly important.

Caring for a loved one with Alzheimer's can be a challenging and demanding experience, but it can also be an opportunity for personal growth and development. By finding ways to prioritize self-care, strengthen relationships, and appreciate the present moment, caregivers can find the silver lining in this challenging experience.

Paying it Forward and Raising Awareness

Caring for a loved one with Alzheimer's can be a challenging and demanding experience. Still, it can also be an opportunity to pay it forward and raise awareness about the disease. Here are a few ways to support others and raise awareness about Alzheimer's:

1. **Share Your Story:**

Sharing your caregiving journey with others can be a powerful way to raise awareness about Alzheimer's and connect with others going through a similar experience. Sharing your story can be done through writing, speaking, or sharing on social media.

2. **Volunteer:**

Many organizations support individuals with Alzheimer's and their caregivers, and volunteering with one of these organizations can be a meaningful way to give back.

3. **Donate:**

Donating to organizations that support individuals with Alzheimer's and their caregivers is a simple but impactful way to help others.

4. **Educate Yourself:**

Learning about Alzheimer's and staying up-to-date on the latest research and developments can help you better understand the disease and how to support loved ones with Alzheimer's.

5. **Raise Awareness:**

There are many ways to raise awareness about Alzheimer's, such as participating in a walk or event, wearing a ribbon, or sharing information about the disease on social media.

Caring for a loved one with Alzheimer's can be a challenging and demanding experience. Still, it can also be an opportunity to pay it forward and raise awareness about the disease.

By sharing your story, volunteering, donating, educating yourself, and raising awareness, you can positively impact the lives of others affected by Alzheimer's.

Advances in Alzheimer's Research and Treatment

Alzheimer's disease is a complex and devastating condition, but researchers and scientists worldwide are working tirelessly to understand the disease better and develop new treatments.

Here are a few exciting advances in Alzheimer's research and treatment:

1. **Early Detection:**

Researchers are working on developing new tools and techniques for detecting Alzheimer's in its early stages before symptoms start to appear. Early detection is critical for improving treatment outcomes and for allowing individuals with Alzheimer have to plan for the future.

2. **Biomarkers:**

Researchers are also working on identifying biomarkers for Alzheimer's, which are specific changes in the body that can indicate the presence of the disease. Identifying biomarkers can help with early diagnosis and monitoring treatments' effectiveness.

3. **Novel Therapies:**

Scientists are developing new therapies for Alzheimer's that target the underlying causes of the disease rather than just managing symptoms. These therapies may include medications, vaccines, and other interventions.

4. **Caregiver Support:**

Researchers are also focusing on developing interventions and support programs to help caregivers manage the demands of caring for a loved one with Alzheimer's.

While there is still much work to be done, these advances in Alzheimer's research and treatment offer hope for the future and the possibility of improved outcomes for individuals with Alzheimer's and their caregivers.

Chapter 7

What are Causes of Alzheimer's?

Alzheimer's is a complex disorder caused by genetic, environmental, and lifestyle factors. Researchers have been studying the causes of Alzheimer's for decades, but there is still much that is not fully understood about this disease.

Below are some of the factors that are believed to contribute to the development of Alzheimer's:

1. **Genetics:**

While most Alzheimer's cases are not directly inherited, specific genes that increase the risk of developing the disease have been identified. The most well-known of these genes is the APOE gene, which comes in different forms (alleles).

The presence of the APOE4 allele is associated with an increased risk of developing Alzheimer's, but having the APOE2 allele may lower the risk.

2. **Age:**

Advancing age is one of the most decisive risk factors for Alzheimer's disease. The risk of developing the disease doubles approximately every five years after age 65.

3. **Environmental Factors:**

Some environmental factors, such as exposure to toxins or head injuries, may increase the risk of developing Alzheimer's disease. Studies have also suggested a possible link between air pollution and Alzheimer's.

4. **Lifestyle Factors:**

Certain lifestyle factors, such as lack of physical exercise, poor diet, smoking, and social isolation, may increase the risk of developing Alzheimer's disease.

5. **Abnormal Protein Accumulation:**

Beta-amyloid plaques and tau tangles are two aberrant proteins that build up in the brain as a result of Alzheimer's disease. These proteins disrupt the normal functioning of brain cells and lead to their death.

6. **Neuroinflammation:**

Neuroinflammation is a process by which the immune system responds to injury or infection in the brain. Chronic neuroinflammation may contribute to the development of Alzheimer's disease.

It's important to note that while these factors are believed to contribute to the development of Alzheimer's, not everyone who has these risk factors will develop the disease. Additionally, there may be other factors that contribute to the development of Alzheimer's that are not yet fully understood.

What Are The Different Stages Of Alzheimer's?

Alzheimer's disease is a degenerative brain condition that impairs cognition and causes memory loss. Alzheimer's disease progresses through three stages: early, medium, and late.

As the disease advances, each stage is distinguished by a unique combination of symptoms that might help family members and caregivers prepare.

Early Stage:

A person may exhibit modest cognitive impairment in the early stages of Alzheimer's, such as forgetfulness and attention problems. They could need help with routine activities like handling money or operating a vehicle. The symptoms of this stage may be so mild that they go unnoticed for several years.

Middle Stage:

As Alzheimer's disease worsens, it moves into this stage. A person's symptoms grow more overt and evident throughout this stage. They could struggle with daily tasks like bathing and dressing, experience personality changes, and have trouble speaking and communicating. A person may need greater help and support from carers throughout this stage, which can extend for several years.

Late Stage:

In the ultimate stage of Alzheimer's, a person may experience severe symptoms, including complete loss of physical and verbal abilities. All facets of daily life, like eating and using the restroom, may require assistance. During this stage, which can persist for many months to several years, a person might need 24-hour care.

Bottom Line

Remember that not every person with Alzheimer's will go through these stages at the same rate or in the same fashion. The rate of the disease's progression varies significantly from person to person; some may quickly deteriorate while others may endure prolonged stability. Caregivers and loved ones can create an individualized care plan that considers a person's particular requirements and preferences in collaboration with medical specialists.

What Are The Warning Signs Of Alzheimer's Disease?

Alzheimer's is a neurodegenerative disorder affecting the brain, causing memory loss and cognitive decline. The disease usually progresses slowly over several years, and early detection can help individuals and families prepare for the future.

Here are some of the common warning signs of Alzheimer's disease:

1. Memory Loss That Disrupts Daily Life:

One of the most common signs of Alzheimer's is memory loss, especially forgetting important dates or events. Individuals with Alzheimer's may also repeatedly ask for the same information, rely on memory aids or family members for things they used to handle on their own, and forget conversations they just had.

2. Difficulty Planning or Solving Problems:

Alzheimer's can cause individuals to have difficulty planning or completing familiar tasks, such as following a recipe or balancing a checkbook. They may also need help concentrating or taking longer to complete tasks than usual.

3. **Challenges with Familiar Tasks:**

Individuals with Alzheimer's may have trouble performing familiar tasks, like driving to a familiar location or managing finances. They may also need help remembering how to play a favorite game or prepare a meal.

4. **Confusion with Time or Place:**

Individuals with Alzheimer's may lose track of dates, seasons, or the passage of time. They may also need to remember where or how they got there.

5. **Problems with Speaking or Writing:**

Alzheimer's can cause individuals difficulty finding the right words or following a conversation. They may also need help with vocabulary, have trouble naming familiar objects, or repeat themselves frequently.

6. Poor Judgment or Decision-Making:

Alzheimer's can cause individuals to have poor judgment, such as giving large sums of money to telemarketers. They may also need to make better decisions when it comes to personal hygiene, such as neglecting to bathe or wear appropriate clothing.

7. Social Withdrawal:

Alzheimer's can cause individuals to withdraw from social activities, hobbies, and other interests. They may also need help keeping up with a favorite sports team or following a favorite television show.

Conclusion

It's important to note that not everyone with Alzheimer's will experience all of these warning signs; some may experience them at different times and in different ways. If you or a loved one is experiencing any warning signs, it's essential to consult a healthcare professional for a thorough evaluation.

Chapter 8

Is There A Cure For Alzheimer's?

Alzheimer's disease is a complex disorder that affects millions of people worldwide. Despite ongoing research, there is currently no cure for Alzheimer's. However, some treatments can help manage the disease's symptoms and improve the quality of life for those affected.

Here are some key points to keep in mind when discussing the search for a cure for Alzheimer's:

1. Current Treatments:

There are medications available that can help manage the symptoms of Alzheimer's, such as memory loss and confusion. These drugs function by raising the concentrations of specific neurotransmitters in the brain.

2. Research on Potential Treatments:

There are many ongoing clinical trials to develop new treatments for Alzheimer's. These treatments include drugs that target beta-amyloid and tau proteins, which are believed to play a role in the development of the disease.

Other potential treatments include immunotherapy, stem cell therapy, and gene therapy.

3. Challenges in Finding A Cure:

Developing a cure for Alzheimer's is a complex process that involves understanding the underlying mechanisms of the disease. One of the challenges in developing a cure is that Alzheimer's is a progressive disease, meaning that symptoms worsen over time.

Finding a cure makes it challenging to develop treatments that can slow or reverse the course of the disease. Additionally, Alzheimer's is a multifactorial disease, which involves a combination of genetic, environmental, and lifestyle factors, making it difficult to target with a single treatment.

4. Promising Research:

Despite the challenges, there are some promising avenues of research in the search for a cure for Alzheimer's. For example, research has shown that lifestyle factors such as exercise and diet may play a role in preventing or slowing disease progression. Additionally, advances in technology, such as brain imaging and biomarkers, are helping researchers better understand the underlying mechanisms of Alzheimer's and identify potential targets for treatment.

In conclusion, while there is currently no cure for Alzheimer's, ongoing research provides hope for the future. By better understanding the underlying mechanisms of the disease and developing new treatments, researchers hope to one day find a cure for this devastating disorder.

What Is The Main Problem With Alzheimer's Disease?

Alzheimer's disease is a progressive brain disorder that causes a gradual decline in cognitive function, including memory, thinking, and reasoning skills. The main problem in Alzheimer's disease is the accumulation of abnormal proteins in the brain, leading to brain cell death and the progressive deterioration of cognitive function.

Here are some key points to keep in mind when discussing the main problem of Alzheimer's disease:

1. **Beta-amyloid**: One of the main abnormal proteins that accumulate in the brains of people with Alzheimer's disease is beta-amyloid. Beta-amyloid produces sticky plaques between neurons that obstruct communication and lead to the death of brain cells.

2. **Tau Protein**: Another abnormal protein that accumulates in the brains of people with Alzheimer's disease is tau protein. Tau protein forms a tangle within neurons, which disrupts

their ability to transport nutrients and other essential molecules throughout the brain.

3. **Neuroinflammation**: Neuroinflammation is another feature of Alzheimer's disease besides the buildup of aberrant proteins. Neuroinflammation is the brain's response to the accumulation of abnormal proteins, which leads to the activation of immune cells and the release of inflammatory molecules.

Over time, chronic neuroinflammation can lead to the death of brain cells and further cognitive decline.

4. **Vascular Changes**: Some research has suggested that vascular changes, such as reduced blood flow to the brain, may also play a role in the development of Alzheimer's disease. These changes can lead to the death of brain cells and contribute to cognitive decline.

In conclusion, the main problem in Alzheimer's disease is the accumulation of abnormal proteins in the brain, leading to brain cell death and the progressive deterioration of cognitive function. While the exact cause of this accumulation is not fully understood, ongoing research is providing new insights into the disease's underlying mechanisms and identifying potential treatment targets.

Can Alzheimer's Be Prevented?

While there is no known cure for Alzheimer's disease, there are some steps that individuals can take to reduce their risk of developing the condition.

While no single measure can guarantee prevention, adopting a healthy lifestyle can reduce the risk of developing Alzheimer's disease.

Here are some strategies for lowering the risk of Alzheimer's:

1. Exercise Regularly:

Studies have shown that regular exercise can reduce the risk of developing Alzheimer's disease by up to 50%. Physical activity can help reduce inflammation and improve circulation, vital for brain health.

2. Follow A Healthy Diet:

A healthy diet rich in fruits, vegetables, whole grains, lean protein, and healthy fats is often associated with a reduced risk of Alzheimer's disease. It is also recommended to limit the intake of processed foods, sugar, and saturated fats.

3. Maintain A Healthy Weight:

Obesity has been linked to an increased risk of developing Alzheimer's disease. This risk can be decreased by maintaining a healthy weight with a balanced diet and regular exercise.

4. Manage Blood Pressure, Cholesterol, And Blood Sugar Levels:

High blood pressure, high cholesterol, and high blood sugar levels are associated with an increased risk of Alzheimer's disease. Managing these factors through lifestyle changes and, if necessary, medication can help reduce the risk of developing the condition.

5. Stay Mentally Active:

Engaging in mentally stimulating activities, such as reading, doing crossword puzzles, or learning a new skill, has reduced the risk of

Alzheimer's disease. These activities help keep the brain active and may promote the growth of new brain cells.

6. Socialize Regularly:

Maintaining social connections has been associated with a reduced risk of Alzheimer's disease. Social interaction helps relieve stress, which can contribute to cognitive decline.

Conclusion

While these measures may not guarantee the prevention of Alzheimer's disease, they can help reduce the risk of developing the condition. It is important to note that some risk factors, such as genetics and age, cannot be controlled. However, by adopting a healthy lifestyle, individuals can take steps to reduce their risk and promote overall health and well-being.

Chapter 9

How Long Does Alzheimers Last?

Alzheimer's disease is a degenerative brain condition that decreases cognitive performance over time. Alzheimer's disease is a fatal ailment, and there is no cure for it. The typical survival time after the onset of symptoms is between 8 and 10 years.

However, the disease's course varies greatly from person to person and can extend for many years. Nevertheless, some individuals may have Alzheimer's for up to 20 years.

Age, general health, and the stage of the disease at which it is identified are some variables that affect how long Alzheimer's disease lasts. Alzheimer's disease symptoms develop from mild to severe over time.

As the disease progresses, the symptoms may become more severe, including memory loss, disorientation, and difficulties carrying out daily chores. In the early stages, the symptoms may be moderate and hardly detectable. Later on, the patient can end up reliant on others for care.

Alzheimer's disease has no known cure. However, medication can help manage the symptoms and enhance the quality of life for those with the condition. Early detection of Alzheimer's disease is crucial because it can be treated and managed more effectively and with slowed disease progression.

Bottom Line

In conclusion, the period that a person with Alzheimer's disease survives might differ from person to person and ranges from 8 to 10 years on average. However, some individuals may endure the illness for up to 20 years. Alzheimer's disease has no known cure, but early detection and treatment can help manage symptoms and enhance prognosis.

Strategies for Preventing Alzheimer

While there is no surefire way to prevent Alzheimer's disease, there are several lifestyle changes and habits that you can adopt to reduce your risk of developing the disease.

Here are some vital strategies that may help prevent alzheimer:

1. Exercise Regularly:

Studies have shown that physical activity can help reduce the risk of Alzheimer's disease. Regular exercise can help improve blood flow to the brain, reduce inflammation, and promote the growth of new brain cells. Attempt to engage in moderate-intensity exercise most days of the week for at least 30 minutes.

2. Follow A Healthy Diet:

A diet rich in fruits, vegetables, whole grains, lean protein, and healthy fats can help reduce the risk of Alzheimer's disease. Steer clear of processed foods, sweetened beverages, and saturated and trans fats.

3. Stay Mentally Active:

Engage in activities stimulating your brain, such as reading, puzzles, and games. Studies have shown that mentally stimulating activities can help build up cognitive reserves, which may delay the onset of Alzheimer's disease.

4. Get Enough Sleep:

Poor sleep quality and quantity have been linked to an increased risk of Alzheimer's disease. Set a goal of 7-8 hours of sleep each night and adopt appropriate sleeping habits.

5. Manage Chronic Health Conditions:

Chronic health conditions such as high blood pressure, diabetes, and obesity have been linked to an increased risk of Alzheimer's disease. Manage these conditions through healthy lifestyle habits, such as exercise and a healthy diet, and follow your doctor's treatment plan.

6. Socialize:

Alzheimer's disease risk has been linked to social isolation and loneliness. Stay connected with friends and family, and engages in social activities that you enjoy.

While there is no guaranteed way to prevent Alzheimer's, adopting healthy lifestyle habits and following these strategies can help reduce your risk of developing the disease. It's always possible to start changing your lifestyle and taking steps to protect your brain health.

Is Alzheimer's Genetic?

Alzheimer's disease is a complex condition that various factors, including genetics, environment, and lifestyle, can cause. While it is not entirely clear what causes Alzheimer's disease, genetics plays a role in its development. According to the Alzheimer's Association, about 1% of all cases of Alzheimer's disease are caused by genetic mutations, which can be passed down through families.

Genetic factors do not directly cause the majority of Alzheimer's cases. However, having a family history of Alzheimer's can increase the risk of developing the disease.

Research suggests that if a parent or sibling has had Alzheimer's disease, an individual's risk of developing the disease is two to three times higher than someone who does not have a family history of the disease.

It is important to note that having a genetic predisposition to Alzheimer's does not mean a person will develop the disease. Many other factors, such as lifestyle and environment, can also contribute to the development of Alzheimer's disease.

Conclusion

In summary, while genetics does play a role in the development of Alzheimer's disease, it is not the only factor. A family history of the disease can increase the risk of developing Alzheimer's, but lifestyle changes and other preventative measures can also help reduce the risk.

Chapter 10

How Does Alzheimer's Begin?

Alzheimer's disease is a progressive brain ailment that gradually impairs thinking and memory abilities, eventually making it unable to carry out daily tasks. While the exact cause of Alzheimer's disease is not fully understood, researchers believe that a combination of genetic, environmental, and lifestyle factors causes it.

The first signs of Alzheimer's disease often involve memory lapses, particularly of recent events. As the disease progresses, other symptoms may develop, including difficulty with language, mood swings, disorientation, and behavioral changes. These symptoms can vary from person to person, and the progression of the disease can be slow or rapid.

At the cellular level, Alzheimer's disease is characterized by accumulating two abnormal proteins in the brain: beta-amyloid and tau. Beta-amyloid protein clumps together to form plaques that can disrupt communication between brain cells.

Tau protein forms a tangle that can disturb the internal support structure of brain cells, leading to their eventual death. These changes can begin years before any symptoms of Alzheimer's disease appear.

Research has also suggested that inflammation and oxidative stress may play a role in the development of Alzheimer's disease. Inflammation occurs when the immune system responds to injury or infection, and chronic inflammation has been linked to a range of chronic diseases, including Alzheimer's. An imbalance between free radicals and antioxidants in the body leads to oxidative stress, which can harm cells.

Bottom Line

In conclusion, Alzheimer's disease begins with the accumulation of abnormal proteins in the brain, which can disrupt communication between brain cells and lead to their eventual death.

While the exact cause of Alzheimer's disease is not fully understood, researchers believe that a combination of genetic, environmental, and lifestyle factors may contribute to its development.

Who Is Likely To Get Alzheimer's?

Alzheimer's is a complex disease; while anyone can develop it, some people may be more at risk than others. The most significant risk factor for Alzheimer's is age, and the risk increases as people get older.

According to the Alzheimer's Association, after age 65, the risk of developing Alzheimer's doubles every five years. By age 85, the risk of Alzheimer's is almost 50%.

Certain genetic factors may increase the risk of developing Alzheimer's disease. Two types of genes are associated with Alzheimer's disease: risk genes and deterministic genes. Risk genes increase the likelihood of developing Alzheimer's but do not guarantee it will happen.

The apolipoprotein E (APOE) ε4 allele is the most common risk gene. Alzheimer's disease risk increases with the number of copies of the

4 allele inherited, with two copies increasing risk even further.

Deterministic genes, on the other hand, directly cause a person to develop Alzheimer's disease, and they are very rare. One example of a deterministic gene is the APP gene, which causes a rare Alzheimer's disease called early-onset familial Alzheimer's disease (EOFAD).

Other factors that may increase the risk of Alzheimer's include lifestyle and environmental factors. These factors include a sedentary lifestyle, a diet high in saturated and trans fats, smoking, high blood pressure, high cholesterol, and head injuries.

It's important to note that just because someone has one or more risk factors doesn't necessarily mean they will develop Alzheimer's. Conversely, someone without these risk factors can still develop the disease.

Although there is currently no method to accurately predict who will get Alzheimer's, knowing the risk factors might help people take precautions to lower their risk and perhaps delay or prevent the disease's start.

What Triggers People with Alzheimer's?

Alzheimer's is a complex disease that affects people differently, making it difficult to pinpoint specific triggers. However, certain factors can contribute to the development and progression of Alzheimer's disease.

There is no denying that Alzheimer's is a terrible disease, whether you are dealing with it yourself or are watching a loved one live with it. Additionally, as more researchers investigate potential illness triggers, they find increasing evidence linking common exposures to an elevated risk. Although no study has yet conclusively stated, "Yes, this is what causes Alzheimer's," these five factors are thought to contribute to the disease and should be avoided.

1. Depression

Even when it comes to dementia and Alzheimer's disease, it is undeniable that our minds and bodies are intertwined. In a groundbreaking 2010 study, it was found that for every ten-point increase in depression scores at the beginning of the trial, the chance of dementia increased by 50%.

Similar hazards existed for Alzheimer's disease, with a 40% risk rise for every 10 points higher depression scores. People with depression were 1.5 times more likely than non-depressed people to have either dementia or Alzheimer's disease.

2. Negative Thoughts

According to Yale experts, Alzheimer's disease is probably influenced by your mindset. Negative stereotypes of aging, such as the idea that older people are "decrepit," have been connected to Alzheimer's disease-related brain abnormalities. Stress brought on by the unfavorable stereotypes about aging that people occasionally internalize from society might cause pathological brain changes.

Even if the results are alarming, it is heartening to know that these unfavorable ideas about aging can be lessened and positive beliefs about aging can be strengthened, such that the negative impact is not unavoidable.

3. Common Medications

Recent studies published in JAMA Internal Medicine found a connection between dementia and Alzheimer's disease and common drugs, including antidepressants and over-the-counter antihistamines. Anticholinergic medicines are those in the issue. These medicines include over-the-counter diphenhydramine, first-generation antihistamines like chlorpheniramine, tricyclic antidepressants like doxepin (Sinequan), and antimuscarinics for bladder control like oxybutynin.

The data also imply that the effects may not be reversible, even after you stop using the drug. The researchers discovered that these effects are dosage dependent (the more anticholinergic medication you take, the higher your chance of getting dementia).

4. DDT

A 2014 study found that higher blood levels of DDE, a toxic insecticide DDT's breakdown component, appeared to exacerbate

Alzheimer's disease. If more research confirms those results, it might imply that screening for DDE levels in the body could result in an earlier diagnosis, which has been found to lessen Alzheimer's symptoms.

Although DDT has been prohibited in the US since 1972, it is used there, and disposal sites can release DDE and other breakdown products into the environment. According to the Centers for Disease Control and Prevention, meat, poultry, dairy products, and fish, mainly sport fish, make up most of a person's daily intake of DDT.

5. Lead

Lead poses a concern to adults as well as kids. Adults with high blood lead levels had an increased chance of developing dementia, according to a 2009 study. 21% of those with above-average lead had results that suggested mild cognitive impairment. Additionally, those with high blood pressure, a risk factor for dementia, tended to have higher levels of lead in their bodies.

According to earlier studies, older persons with high lead levels are at an increased risk for cardiovascular disease. Lead can raise inflammation in the body, producing oxidative stress on the brain and rising blood pressure.

If you live in a home built before 1978, you should get the interior and exterior paint in your home lead-tested and avoid using vinyl items.

Lost and Found

Chapter 11

What Is The Best Treatment For Alzheimer?

Alzheimer's disease, a progressive neurodegenerative disorder, affects memory, thinking, and behavior. There is currently no cure for Alzheimer's disease, and the available treatments aim to manage the symptoms and improve the quality of life for individuals with the disease.

The best treatment for Alzheimer's depends on the disease's stage and the individual's specific symptoms. Treatment options may include medications, lifestyle changes, and support services.

Medications that are commonly used to treat Alzheimer's disease include cholinesterase inhibitors and memantine. These medications can help improve cognitive symptoms, such as memory loss, and may also help with behavioral symptoms. However, these medications do not stop the progression of the disease and may only provide temporary benefits.

In addition to medications, lifestyle changes can also benefit individuals with Alzheimer's disease. Regular exercise, a healthy diet, and social engagement have all been shown to improve cognitive function and reduce the risk of cognitive decline.

Caregiver support services, such as respite care and support groups, can also help manage the emotional and practical challenges of caring for a loved one with Alzheimer's.

It's important to note that there is no one-size-fits-all approach to treating Alzheimer's disease, and the best treatment plan will depend on the individual's unique situation. Each individual will require a different treatment plan, which a healthcare professional can determine.

To temporarily alleviate some symptoms of Alzheimer's disease, you can use a variety of medications. The primary medicines are:

1. **Acetylcholinesterase (AChE) inhibitors**

These medications produce acetylcholine, a chemical that facilitates nerve cell communication in the brain, in greater quantities. Currently, only professionals like psychiatrists or neurologists are permitted to prescribe them.

They may be recommended by a general practitioner (GP) who has specific knowledge of their use or on the advice of a specialist.

For those with early- to mid-stage Alzheimer's disease, doctors may prescribe donepezil, galantamine, and rivastigmine. The most recent recommendations advise continuing these medications into the disease's later, more severe phases.

Each of the three AChE inhibitors works equally well. Still, some people react better to one type than another or experience fewer side effects, including nausea, vomiting, and appetite loss. Usually, adverse effects subside after two weeks of pharmaceutical use.

2. Memantine

There is no AChE inhibitor in this medication. It obstructs the effects of too much glutamate, a neurotransmitter in the brain. For Alzheimer's disease that is moderate to severe, memantine is prescribed. It is appropriate for people who cannot tolerate or use AChE inhibitors.

Additionally, it is appropriate for those currently on an AChE inhibitor and with severe Alzheimer's disease. Headaches, lightheadedness, and constipation are possible side effects; however, they are typically relatively transient. Read the patient information leaflet with your medication or consult your doctor for more details regarding any potential side effects.

Bottom Line

While there is no cure for Alzheimer's, a combination of medication, lifestyle changes, and support services can help manage the symptoms and improve the quality of life for individuals with the disease.

What Organ Does Alzheimer's Disease Affect?

Alzheimer's disease primarily affects the brain and gradually causes the brain cells to degenerate and die, leading to a decline in cognitive function and memory loss. Specifically, Alzheimer's disease affects the cerebral cortex, the part of the brain responsible for thought, memory, and language.

As the disease progresses, other brain areas, such as the hippocampus, which is essential for memory formation, also become affected.

The brain shrinks in size, and protein deposits called beta-amyloid plaques and tau tangles replace the brain tissue. These plaques and tangles interfere with the communication between the brain cells, leading to cognitive and memory impairment observed in Alzheimer's patients.

What Foods Reduce Alzheimer's?

Alzheimer's is a complex disease that currently has no cure. Still, some evidence suggests that a healthy diet can help reduce the risk of developing the disease and potentially slow its progression in those who already have it. Here are some foods that may have a positive effect on Alzheimer's:

1. **Fatty Fish**: Fish like salmon, mackerel, and sardines are high in omega-3 fatty acids, which are linked to a reduced risk of Alzheimer's disease.
2. **Berries**: Blueberries, strawberries, and blackberries are rich in antioxidants and may help protect brain cells from damage.
3. **Leafy Greens**: Dark, leafy greens like spinach, kale, and collard greens are packed with nutrients like vitamin E and folate, which may help protect against Alzheimer's.

4. **Nuts**: Almonds, walnuts, and hazelnuts are high in vitamin E and healthy fats, which may help protect against cognitive decline.
5. **Whole Grains**: Whole grains like brown rice, oatmeal, and quinoa contain nutrients like vitamin E, folate, and fiber, which have been linked to a reduced risk of Alzheimer's disease.

It's important to note that while these foods may be beneficial, a healthy diet alone is not enough to prevent or cure Alzheimer's. Keeping a healthy weight, exercising regularly, and avoiding smoking and excessive alcohol consumption are also important.

Chapter 12

Has Anyone Ever Recovered From Alzheimer's?

Alzheimer's disease is a progressive disease that currently has no cure. However, treatments available can slow the disease's progression and improve the quality of life for those living with it. Unfortunately, no one has ever fully recovered from Alzheimer's disease.

While there is no cure for Alzheimer's, research is ongoing to find ways to prevent or treat the disease. Some studies have shown promising results with treatments to slow the disease's progression or target specific symptoms. For example, a study published in the journal Science Translational Medicine found that a drug called "NTRX-07" showed promise in reducing inflammation in the brains of mice with Alzheimer's disease. However, more research is needed to determine if this treatment will be effective in humans.

It is also worth noting that there have been cases where individuals with symptoms of dementia, including Alzheimer's, have been misdiagnosed. Sometimes, the symptoms may have been caused by treatable conditions such as depression, medication side effects, or vitamin deficiencies. In these cases, appropriate treatment can significantly improve cognitive function.

What's The Difference Between Alzheimer's And Dementia?

Alzheimer's disease and dementia are two terms often used interchangeably, but they are not the same. Dementia is an umbrella term that refers to symptoms associated with a decline in cognitive functioning, including memory loss, difficulty with language and communication, and problems with reasoning and judgment. Alzheimer's disease is a specific type of dementia, accounting for 60-80% of dementia cases.

One of the main differences between Alzheimer's disease and other forms of dementia is that Alzheimer's is a progressive disease, which means that it gets worse over time.

Alzheimer's disease specifically affects the brain's ability to form and retain memories and carry out basic cognitive tasks such as making decisions or performing familiar tasks. As the disease progresses, it can also affect a person's personality, behavior, and communication ability.

Dementia, conversely, is a more general term encompassing a range of conditions that cause cognitive decline. In addition to Alzheimer's, there are several other types of dementia, including vascular dementia, Lewy body dementia, and frontotemporal dementia.

Each of these conditions has its own unique set of symptoms and causes and may progress at different rates.

Has Anyone Ever Survived Alzheimer's Disease?

Unfortunately, Alzheimer's is a progressive and irreversible condition with no cure. While there are treatments available that can slow the progression of the disease and manage symptoms, there is no known way to reverse the damage caused by Alzheimer's entirely.

In other words, no known case exists of someone completely recovering from Alzheimer's. However, it's important to note that people with Alzheimer's can live for many years after their diagnosis.

With the proper treatment and support, they can maintain a good quality of life for as long as possible. Additionally, ongoing research is being conducted into potential treatments and cures for Alzheimer's, giving hope for future breakthroughs and advances.

Chapter 13

How Much Sleep Do You Need To Prevent Alzheimer's?

While no exact number of hours of sleep can prevent Alzheimer's disease, studies suggest that getting adequate and quality sleep can help reduce the risk of developing the disease.

Sleep plays a vital role in maintaining brain function, including the clearance of beta-amyloid protein, a hallmark of Alzheimer's disease. When beta-amyloid accumulates in the brain, it can form plaques that disrupt communication between brain cells and cause inflammation. Chronic sleep deprivation may interfere with this clearance process and increase the risk of developing Alzheimer's disease.

One study found that older adults who reported poor sleep quality or short sleep duration had higher levels of beta-amyloid in their brains than those who slept better. Another study found that individuals who slept less than six hours a night had an increased risk of developing Alzheimer's.

Therefore, it is recommended that adults aim for 7-8 hours of sleep each night to maintain optimal brain function and potentially reduce the risk of Alzheimer's disease.

Additionally, practicing good sleep hygiene, such as establishing a consistent bedtime routine, avoiding screens before bedtime, and creating a comfortable sleep environment, may improve sleep quality and reduce the risk of developing Alzheimer's disease.

Do Eggs Prevent Alzheimer's?

While there is no definitive evidence to suggest that eating eggs can prevent Alzheimer's disease, some studies have indicated that specific components of eggs may have potential neuroprotective effects.

Eggs are a good source of choline, a nutrient that plays a role in brain function and has been associated with better cognitive performance and reduced risk of dementia in some studies.

Additionally, eggs contain antioxidants, such as lutein and zeaxanthin, which have been associated with better cognitive function and may help to protect against oxidative stress, which is thought to contribute to Alzheimer's disease.

However, it is essential to note that Alzheimer's disease is a complex condition with multiple risk factors, and no single food or nutrient can guarantee protection against it.

Maintaining a healthy, balanced diet that includes a variety of nutrient-rich foods, such as fruits, vegetables, whole grains, lean proteins, and healthy fats, is generally recommended as part of a lifestyle that may help reduce the risk of Alzheimer's disease and other chronic health conditions.

Additionally, engaging in regular physical activity, managing stress, getting adequate sleep, and staying socially connected are other essential factors that may help promote brain health and reduce the risk of Alzheimer's disease.

How Can I Prevent My Parents From Getting Alzheimer's?

As we age, our risk of developing Alzheimer's disease increases, and it's natural to be concerned about our parents' health. Although there is no guaranteed way to prevent Alzheimer's disease, some lifestyle changes and strategies can reduce the risk of developing the disease.

Here are some steps you can take to help prevent your parents from getting Alzheimer's:

- Encourage them to exercise their bodies frequently. Studies have shown that exercise can help reduce the risk of developing Alzheimer's disease. Even low to moderate-intensity activities, such as walking, can be beneficial.

- Promote a healthy diet of fruits, vegetables, and lean proteins. A Mediterranean-style diet, which includes plenty of vegetables, legumes, fruits, and whole grains, has been linked to a lower risk of Alzheimer's disease.

- Encourage your parents to stay socially engaged. Alzheimer's disease risk has been linked to social exclusion and loneliness. Encourage your parents to participate in social activities such as clubs, volunteering, or community organizations.

- Help them manage their medical conditions. Chronic health conditions such as diabetes, high blood pressure, and high cholesterol have been linked to an increased risk of Alzheimer's disease. Encourage your parents to manage these conditions with medication, diet, and exercise.

- Encourage them to take part in mentally challenging activities. Activities such as reading, doing crossword puzzles, or playing board games can help keep the mind active and reduce the risk of Alzheimer's disease.

It's important to remember that some risk factors for Alzheimer's disease, such as age and genetics, cannot be changed. However, by making these lifestyle changes and encouraging your parents to adopt healthy habits, you can help reduce their risk of developing Alzheimer's disease.

Conclusion

In conclusion, "Lost and Found" has explored the many challenges and emotions that come with caring for a loved one with Alzheimer's. From the early stages of diagnosis to the difficult decisions around end-of-life care, caregivers are faced with a wide range of challenges and emotions. However, as this journey has shown, it is also an opportunity for growth, learning, and finding hope and joy in the small things.

As we look to the future, it is important to recognize the progress that has been made in the field of Alzheimer's research and treatment, and to continue supporting those affected by the disease. Whether through sharing stories, volunteering, donating, or raising awareness, there are many ways to support individuals with Alzheimer's and their caregivers.

Through this journey, we have seen that it is possible to find healing and hope in the midst of difficult circumstances, and to find meaning and purpose in the small things. As caregivers navigate the ups and downs of caring for a loved one with Alzheimer's, it is important to be patient with oneself, to seek out support when needed, and to find joy and hope in the present moment. Thank you for joining us on this journey through Alzheimer's.

THE END